How To Help Your Disabled Child

H Bastawy

ISBN: 9798323210084

Hera Publishing
Leeds
UK

DEDICATION

To every disabled child who needs help;
Your disability is not your fault,
There is hope.

CONTENTS

ABOUT THE AUTHOR

Dr H Bastawy is a Fellow of the British Higher Education Academy and a Fellow of the Royal Anthropological Institute and a former Teaching Fellow in Drama and Postcolonial Literature at the University of Leeds. He completed his interdisciplinary PhD in English and History at Leeds Trinity University and the University of Leeds. He taught English and History at more than ten universities and colleges in the UK and around the world, read and presented papers at many conferences worldwide and he is an outstanding Ofsted-rated educator. He received the John Murray Prize for the distinction of his research in 2015, the Peter Emmerson 2015 Assessor of the Year Award and the SWAPCA Languages and Literatures Award in the US in February 2017 and has published widely on various aspects of English Literature and History. Some of his stories were featured in movies. Alongside his publications, he also works on his art and his music. His rock album, *Supernova*, has attracted worldwide attention, and some of his songs were featured on TV. He is World number 1 in *Academia* worldwide author ranking. WWW.HBastawy.com

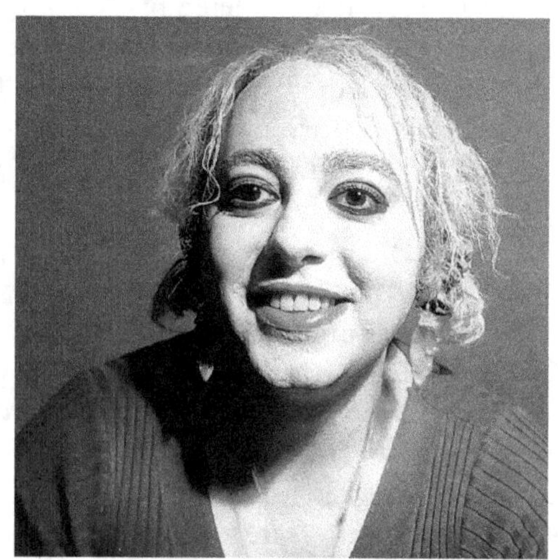

1 INTRODUCTION

'Right Down to Earth in a Language That Everybody Here Understands'

I am Dr H Bastawy. I don't specialize in disabilities or neuro-disabilities. But I have managed through research and experience to help my disabled child who was initially diagnosed with quadruple cerebral palsy – paralysis in all limbs and spine – to eventually develop the ability to stand on his own and take some steps. I thought I would write this as a guide to help anyone who may have a child with difficulties of a similar nature.

At the time of the diagnosis, there was not much movement in his body. And the movements he displayed were very concerning. His back would fall in any direction and when he slept it would arch backwards. There were slight movements in the fingers of his hands and he could feed without difficulties. These were the only positives we had. But they were positives to build on nevertheless. I was told he will never walk or stand on his own, but I did not accept that.

2 BLAME

My disabled child is called Noah. He is a beautiful and lively person who is always looking forward to what he could manage to do next. Considering how severe his disability has been from the beginning, every new step he takes and every new development he makes is a great achievement.

He is twin brother to Aaron. Aaron had other difficulties initially but he managed to overcome them. He could not feed. He had chest problems and he was one third of Noah's weight when he was born. I had to deal with Aaron's difficulties separately when he was born and we eventually managed to sort them out. It is very ironic to me now, that it was Aaron whom I was given the option to terminate during a very complicated pregnancy. Obviously, I rejected. Aaron, unfortunately, continues to have chest problems now. And he is the one prone to coughs and chest colds because of his initial problems.

The pregnancy was a very complicated one, with haemorrhage and bleeding throughout. It did not help that his mother, who is no longer with us – she was practically classed as dead or non-existent to us after their birth -, had drug problems and addictions she could not cope with. The children suffered massively because of that. Drugs fry an adult's brain, you can imagine what they would do to a child that was still being formed. Eventually, they were born very premature. And they struggled to gain normal functions of the lungs for the first few days of their lives.

Noah's disability and Aaron's initial difficulty were largely because of that. The damage this caused, particularly for Noah is something that I will explain in medical terms further on.

I am not however trying to put blame on anyone or anything in particular, but I am putting the disability/injury we have had to deal with within the context that it happened within. Having said that, the same disability could have been caused by any and many reasons which could be, in other situations, be beyond human intervention.

And I am hoping by writing this honest guide to help anyone who may have had to incur such difficulties for any reason within or beyond their reach.

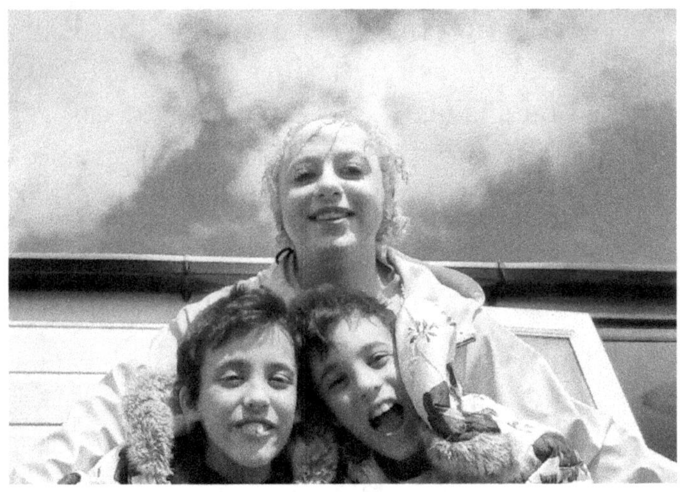

3 BRAIN

Most often the damage caused that leads to this disability is referred to as a damage within the brain. This is not actually the case. The damage/injury that this disability is usually the outcome of happens in an organ that is located underneath the brain, and right above the spine. Not the brain itself.

This organ is called the cerebellum. Hence the name of the disability, cerebral palsy.

In fact, the brain stays completely intact and unaffected.

The figure below shows where the cerebellum is located, which is right under the brain and above the spine in the back of the head.

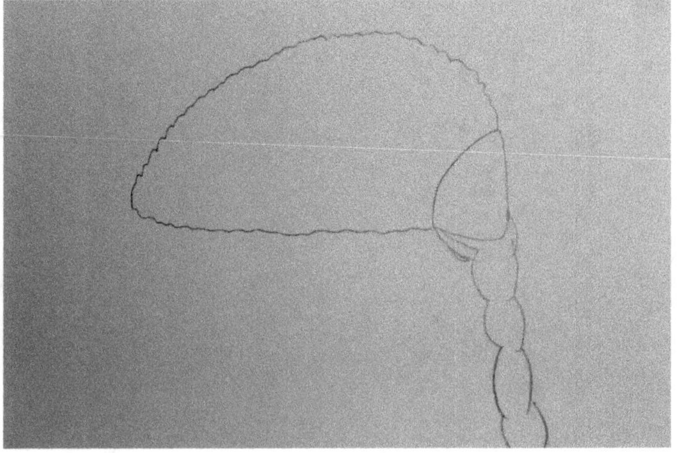

The figure below shows a back view of the cerebellum.

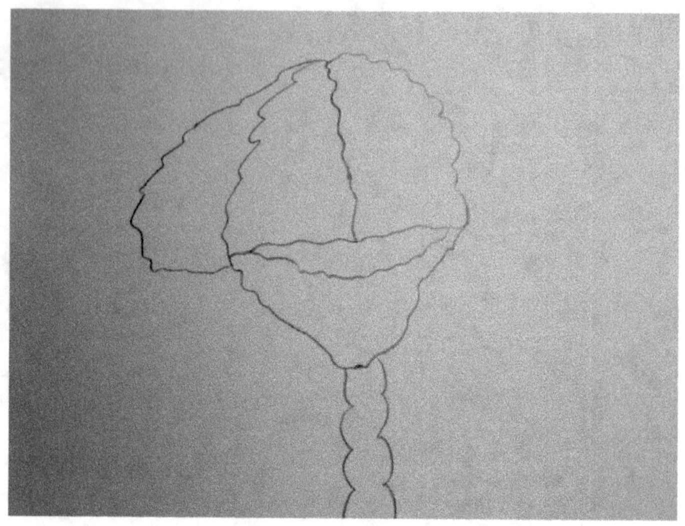

4 MIRACLES BEYOND MEDICINE

The cerebellum as an organ functions as a connector of signals between the brain and the spine. Signals that humans don't think about. Every time a human moves any part of their body, it is down to the communication of signals between the brain and the spine which is conducted through the cerebellum.

The damage that causes the disability that is referred to as cerebral palsy, which means the lack of control of signals of movements between the brain and the spine, and from there to the body, is made of scar tissue.

In this sense, any type of cerebral disability

does not indicate a problem with the body or the brain but a damage within the cerebellum itself where the scar tissue had formed and blocked the signals of communication of movement.

Dealing with the cerebellum itself, where the damage is located, one realized that regardless of what level of damage incurred there would still be large areas left unaffected.

The miracles beyond medicine here then is in these areas and in the nature of the cerebellum as a mass conductor of electric signals between the brain and spine that would always contain loads of spare tissue regardless of how much scar tissue (damaged areas) it incurred.

That's where we found a way forward.

We just simply had to create new connections within the cerebellum, using the spare tissue it contained, for the signals between the brain and the spine, and consequently the body.

We had no case studies of this ever happening before for a child who had never managed to have these signals connected ever before. And we were told that he would never be able to do these things.

But we had our research which was rooted in scientific facts, and we had our belief that our theory could be put into practice. And that was our building foundation for what we managed to achieve.

5 FEEDING

The situation we were in considering the difficulties both twins were having may sound catastrophic. It was definitely difficult but we were focusing on the positives while trying to structure a method of dealing with all of this effectively.

After more than two months in hospital with all attempts of getting him to feed, it had become apparent that it was not going to happen in this environment. Noah had been discharged a month earlier. I asked for Aaron to be discharged too while dealing with his feeding difficulties at home. It was not viable managing a twin at home and a twin at hospital. I had to have both of them with me.

Despite all these problems, Aaron's discharging from hospital was a day of celebration. No more daily trips to the hospital and no more hospital food. They discharged him with loads of packages of tubes and tube-feeding equipment to last for months. The nurses and the doctors had tried everything with him and failed.

The feeding tube went from his nose all the way to his stomach, and he was fed through it. I was supposed to changed it for him every now and again, and change the other feeding equipment. He was nearly three months old and there was no sign of him ever feeding on his own.

After celebrating his discharging from hospital. I sat with him and held him in my arms, and started talking to him as if he understood. 'Noah, is really struggling. And what you're doing is not helping me or him. You need to learn to feed properly so that you can get better and stronger.'

He held my hand as if he understood. I pulled his tube out of his stomach through his nose and prepared a bottle for him. He initially pushed it back. But I held it in his mouth. He tried to push it, but couldn't. I kept it in his mouth. He tried to cry but couldn't. I still held it in his mouth.

'You're going to drink this.' I made sure this was not affecting his breathing and that he was not chalking while doing this.

I noticed a gulp.

I pulled it out, to give him a couple of seconds. I understood how difficult this was for him. He had never used his throat muscles before.

I did the same thing again until I noticed another gulp. I gave him a couple of seconds and so on.

It was a gradual process that day, but he managed to learn to drink/feed himself.

6 WEIGHT

Aaron was a third of Noah's weight when he was born and continued to weigh much less than Noah in the first year. But they were both very premature at birth. And they both needed to put on the weight.

We got them premature milk and with this we started adding things to help with their weight. Butter was one of the main things that we added to their warm bottles of milk. And Aaron had to wear an extra shirt to help him with his chest problems.

Eventually they got to a manageable weight like other babies.

7 REFLECTIVE SIGNALLING

While dealing with the problems of feeding and weight, and as the twins started gaining weight comparable to other babies, one could start to notice the discrepancy in movement ability between the twins. Aaron started to learn to crawl slowly. Noah could not even crawl. But somehow he had managed to learn to keep the milk bottle pressed between his hands while feeding. This was a great development for us.

I had started my research a long time before this stage. And by that point, I was starting to gather other information including brain scans, x-rays and so on which provided me with other dimensions to what I was doing.

I eventually came up with the theory which we put into practice. As I explained the nature of the cerebellum previously. It is a mass conductor of signals of movements from the brain to the spine, to the limbs. If you understand how electricity works, it works both ways. And with the nature of any mass conductor of electricity, it has to work both ways. As I explained earlier, our conclusion in regards to the damage/injury incurred, was there would always be a large amount of spare tissue anyway.

If we have spare tissue, a large amount of it, and with the nature of electricity and conductors of electricity as something that could function both ways, then we could get to pass signals through the spare tissue we have got to bypass the blocked signals in the scar tissue.

In order to do this, we had to make new connections through the spare tissue available. And to do this we had to work the signals the other way round. We could generate the signals through the limbs to the brain through the spare tissue, and in doing so getting them to create their new connections within the cerebellum to the brain.

I called this Reflective Signalling.

The signals would be generated by getting the limbs to do the movements that are blocked by the scar tissue. The signals would be conducted through the cerebellum to the brain and in doing so create new connections that would bypass the injured/scared tissue. The signals from the brain to the spine, in their turn, would then be communicated (they would naturally find a way through) via these new connections that we have created for them, completely bypassing the scar tissue. Eventually the injured/scar tissue becomes irrelevant and completely bypassed, as if it was not there.

The figure below shows the injured tissue and how the signals are bypassing it through the spare tissue within the cerebellum.

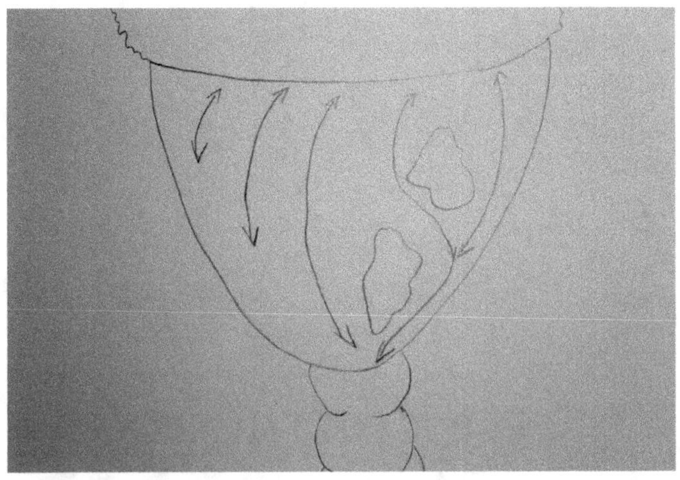

We started with crawling. We put Noah in a crawling position and started to help him make the crawling movements. But neither his arms could support him nor his legs. We persevered. And with daily exercise. Of all limbs. We eventually got there. He was more than two years old by then. That was a long time of trying. But it worked. It eventually worked.

They were just under three years old. Aaron could walk by then, but Noah was getting better at crawling on his own.

From there, we realized that there was no limit to what we could achieve.

8 OUT OF THE PRAM

Until this point, I was using a twins pram to push them around and when needing to go to the shops and so on.

When Aaron started walking, I managed to adapt a baby carrier for Noah that would support his back without him falling backwards.

But now they had outgrown all of that.

Noah had started to crawl, but there was a problem that no body had thought about. He could not sit.

When he would try to sit, his back would collapse on him in any direction. To help him sit after crawling, I would position him with cushions all around him. I even used maternity cushions too.

Our theory of Reflective Signalling worked, but now we needed to create new exercises to create the signals for his muscles of the trunk and the spine.

9 SURGERY

Around that time, we were given the option of surgery.

Surgery is only used in severe cases and that's why it was discussed with us.

There are two types of surgery for these cases: surgery on the cerebellum and surgery on the ligaments.

The surgery on the cerebellum is used to remove as much as possible of the scar/injured tissue which is blocking the signals.

The problem with this is that it is often guess work. Not all the injured tissue is obvious.

And with these areas being so intricate the surgery is very likely to cause damage, or more harm than good. But we were told that it did make some differences in some cases.

The other type of surgery is surgery on the ligaments. Surgery on the ligaments is used to help with the general tightness which is caused by the lack of everyday movements of the limbs.

We rejected both types of surgery. Our Reflective Signalling was working and continues to and it would never cause him harm. And in regards to the ligaments we do several sessions of exercises and stretches everyday anyway as part of our development of his muscle signals.

10 NEW EQUIPMENT

To accommodate for his spine problem, new and customised equipment were needed. Wheel chairs and feeding/everyday chairs needed to be adapted to support the positioning of his back so that it would not collapse on him.

These helped at the time, but they were very unpractical and took too much space. The slightest nudge in any direction, they would damaged tiles and walls. We didn't have time to be fixing things all the time. We were having to fix many things anyway including the children, this was just giving us more things to fix.

Within a couple of years we managed to get

him to a point where he would not need these things and we managed to change them with equipment that was more practical for us. Like a foldable wheelchair that could be used indoors and outdoors for example. It would still support his back but with reinforced cushions rather than a steel frame built around the spine.

Other types of equipment that was discussed was a customised bed to help with his positioning at bedtime. It could also be lowered and raised and would prevent him from falling over in the night.

This deemed itself useless, no bed could prevent his back from collapsing backwards when he slept. And we would have ended up with another thing that would have taken too much space and was very unpractical. Instead we had to continue supporting his back with maternity cushions at bedtime to keep him in good position.

11 ANOTHER WAY AROUND

While looking into all of these, and customising equipment, and looking for equipment and buying equipment and returning equipment, we were looking into a way of developing the signals for the muscles surrounding his spine. This was not something that he could exercise for at this stage yet.

Our way around that was to work on the spine from both directions at the same time. He had developed the ability to crawl and with that the ability to move his limbs to an extent at his will. To work on the spine we were going to do exercises around the areas where he had managed to learn to move them at his will.

In this case, this was going to be the muscles of the shoulders and the back of the shoulders, and the muscles of the legs at the haunches and upwards. This would develop the muscles of the spine in these areas nearer to the limbs, until they are developed enough for us to work on the muscles of his core.

We kept going until he got to a point where he could stand while holding on. He managed to do this by relying mainly on the muscles of the back of his shoulders, some of the muscles of his legs and arms to prevent his back from collapsing. The core area had not been developed at all yet at this stage. We were completely aware of that, but we were making great progress in the areas that we thought he would be able to develop.

12 PARALLEL BARS

It took sometime to find somewhere that manufactured and sold parallel bars for children so young. But that was just what he needed at this point of his development.

I bought them for him and set them up in his room.

The parallel bars as their name suggests are bars opposite each other with a passage in between, and they could be adjusted in height as he grew older.

In principle, the parallel bars and the exercises we would do with them would help him to at least register walking signals.

Now that he could try to stand while holding on for a few seconds. He would hold onto the parallel bars while I held his heels between my toes to do some steps with him.

These movements were movements he had never made in his life and was told he would never do. But everything else he was not supposed to do. He was not going to be able to stand, or crawl, or move his arms, or …

But we were managing to do all these things anyway. It was taking us a long time but it was happening.

Now it was time to walk.

Following the same practices of Reflective Signalling, generating the walking movement signals by moving his legs in the way they were supposed to do had he been able to do that himself, would eventually create the new connections needed for him to do that at his will.

And now that he had developed some movement in his legs by learning to crawl following the same theory and practice over several years, walking was not a far-fetched goal.

We kept doing the parallel bars exercises everyday at least twice, until he got to a point when he could hold onto the bars without me having to hold him at the same time, and we would get to the end of the bars and back.

I was still having to do the walking for him while holding his feet with mine, but he had started to gain some walking movements himself.

Everything took a long time but we eventually got there. Initially, by holding onto one side of the bars and walking side-ways. This way he did not have to carry the full weight of his legs but could shuffle his feet.

And eventually by holding onto the bars properly and walking to the end of them, albeit with great difficulty and by relying mainly on his upper body to prevent his back from collapsing.

The level of strength we had to create in his upper body and the front of his legs to accommodate for the complete trunk paralysis was ridiculous for a child that age and with his severe disability. You could see his muscles on display when he was undressed. But at the same time you could see that there was a part of his body that had not yet been part of our treatment of his cerebral palsy.

We were not far off now. We were closing in on his paralysed core from both directions.

13 EPILEPSY

All children affected by the injury/damage that causes cerebral palsy are very likely to develop epilepsy. This is because of the blocked signals that the brain is trying to send but continue to be blocked by the scar/injured tissue in the cerebellum. These signals end up being bounced back onto the brain, and the more the brain tries to send these signals the more damage is done.

The electric signals that are being blocked by the cerebellum have no way out. In electricity, we call this the earth pole. In this case there is no way of discharging these signals, and they end up bouncing back onto the brain.

And this is very likely to cause epilepsy in addition to cerebral palsy.

Epilepsy is imbalance in the electricity or electric charges of the brain, hence the likelihood of this in cases of cerebral palsy

We were told about this likelihood from the beginning. But nobody seemed to realise why that was a likely scenario for children affected by cerebral palsy.

I came to the conclusion above through my research, which took years.

Reflective Signalling does not eliminate the likelihood of epilepsy for a child affected by cerebral palsy. But it makes it much less likely.

This is because Reflective Signalling creates new connections for the brain to channel its signals through to the spine, and in turn reduces the likelihood of the brain's signals bouncing back on itself which is the ultimate cause of further damage causing epilepsy.

14 WALKING FRAME

The day Noah got his walking frame was a day of celebration for us. And he went in it and walked like he had been doing this before.

Our exercises on the parallel bars had paid off.

We have now reached another level.

He could walk in a walking frame.

15 SETBACKS

Our main setback was not the disability itself, or the injury that caused it. We had already developed an effective theory and practice of treating cerebral palsy.

The main setback was encountering medical professionals who were narrowly specialised in their respective subjects but without any medical background knowledge of the condition itself, or of other things that maybe of relevance.

I had to explain what type of twin Noah and Aaron are so many times in various hospitals. In most occasions the personnel I was talking to had no idea what I was talking about. They were probably brilliant at their subjects but if they don't know anything about the condition itself then they can't really be of any help to my child.

A good example of this is a specialised hospital optician. She did not know what cerebral palsy was and how it was affecting him, but she decided to provide him with a prescription for glasses.

Noah could not see in front of him with these on, he could not read and we were having to read to him. This went on for years and we had appointments with several hospital opticians, one of them was even a consultant.

I even booked an appointment specifically to explain that this could not be right. The prescription he was being provided with was hindering his development. Still, they were not getting what I was saying to them.

Eventually we had to deal with things our way and it worked. He can now read himself without help from anyone. His favourite books are the Polar Bear stories by H Bastawy and Captain Underpants by Dav Pilkey.

16 ACKNOWLEDGEMENT

By mentioning these setbacks, we are not trying to call anybody or point fingers at anybody, we are simply mentioning a problem we had.

We are very grateful to anyone who helped us along the way, professional or not.

But it would have helped, if those who did not know anything about Noah's condition had done some research themselves before trying to offer him help that was really hindering him for years.

We are also aware that our theory and practice of Reflective Signalling which has been proven to treat cerebral palsy is something new and has never been done before. Consequently, what we encountered in terms of the above mentioned setbacks is probably what all children with cerebral palsy encounter everyday.

17 NYSTAGMUS

What the hospital opticians and the consultant opticians were not understanding was that what was affecting Noah was not a problem with his eyes or his sight but something to do with his cerebral palsy which they did not know anything about.

As I explained with how the signals from his brain were affected by the injured/scar tissue, something similar was also happening in this case. Instead of prescribing glasses that he would not see with them on, this was what needed to be looked into. But again there was nothing they could do about it anyway because no way of treating this condition had been developed until we created ours.

The figure below shows the difference between eyes that need help with glasses and what Noah was struggling with and how the very specialised opticians could not tell the difference because both things may appear the same to those who don't know.

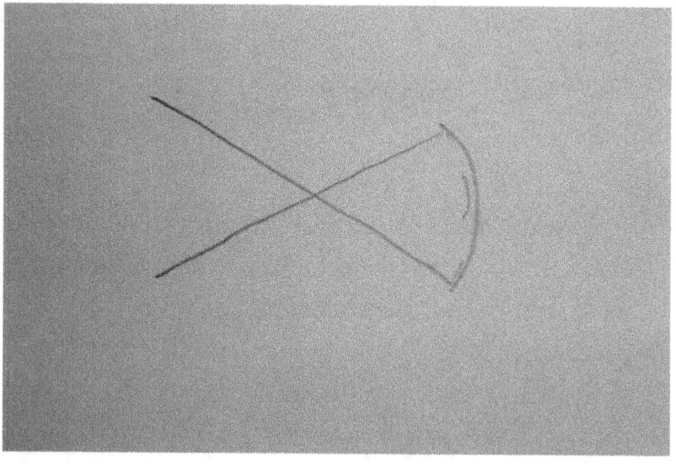

He was in general treated as partially-sighted. One of the many issues the opticians diagnosed him with was something called Nystagmus, pronounced 'Naystagmas'. In this case the person suffering from this problem struggles with fonts, colours, backgrounds and contrasts.

I am trying not to go into very detailed medical information. As I mentioned, my intention from this guide is to help the everyday person help anybody – particularly a child – who has suffered from the injury that caused cerebral palsy. But I will explain this point in simple terms as an example of what we were referring to previously.

Even though this may seem the case and may continue to, Nystagmus is not really what Noah was suffering from but his cerebral palsy itself. For Noah, some faint fonts may not seem very obvious to him. But this has nothing to do with colours or contrasts. It has to do with the way his signals function when he looks at something.

He likes colours. His favourite colour is green. Him and Aaron asked me to paint a rainbow in their room and paint the doorway of the house pink and I did.

Like I said Noah now can read without any help from anybody and without any wrongly-prescribed glasses hindering his development.

He likes to read to me sometimes to show me how good he is at reading, just the way I used to read to him when we had the previous problems.

18 MEDICATION

Children with cerebral palsy can be prescribed many types of medications but for Noah it was mainly a medicine for the tightness of his ligaments.

As I explained in the chapter on the types of surgery offered in these cases. Children with severe cerebral palsy are not expected to be doing much movements, particularly in Noah's case with it being quadruple paralysis of limbs and spine from the beginning.

The medication is supposed to help loosen the ligaments and reduce overall tightness but of course nothing compensates for the actual movements of the limbs themselves.

We did not agree with the dosage prescribed because it would work against what we were aiming to achieve. Overall looseness of ligaments would not support him trying to gain control of his muscles and exercises.

Again, I had to do enough research into the pros and cons of the medication, to see what we could do to help him and at the same time not hinder his development.

The main thing with this type of medication is that it has to be a gradual process when reduced or increased.

We reduced it gradually and tried with him his exercises until we managed to achieve a good balance between his exercise and just enough medication that would support him without hindering his development.

If we were introducing new exercises or stretches, this was something I had to change again gradually until we achieved what was best for him.

The consultant increased the dosage every year based on his age. Eventually, and this was years later, when the consultant realised the significant progress we were making and I explained how I was having to change his dosage to accommodate for his development she left it at our discretion whenever she thought of increasing the dosage.

It was good to have this flexibility with a medical professional who could see what we were achieving with our way of doing things.

19 SPORTS

With walking frames on board, it was time to get Noah to explore different types of exercise from what we were doing every day.

Yes, you guessed it right. We played football.

He could not kick the ball as such but could direct his walking from towards the ball and get the ball to roll in front of him at its impact with his legs.

He was so happy we could all play something like that. Something he often watched from his chairs but could not take part in.

We tried basketball as well from his chair.

It was fun for him to be trying all these new things. It was summer and we had loads and loads of fun.

He even tried swimming with floats and a vest. This is probably the only sport he continued to do after that. He was not much into ball sports.

We have recently tried boxing as well and he had only just managed to learn to punch properly, and he has started to learn to swim without floats. I would say boxing and swimming are the sports he is likely to continue to practice at his wish.

20 THE LAST HURDLE

Despite all our progress in all these areas, there was still part of his body completely paralysed. His core.

We have managed to liberate the upper and lower parts of his spine from this paralysis through the exercises I explained before when we started upright movements in the parallel bars.

But the core was still completely paralysed and his back could still collapse on him in this area. As the figure below shows.

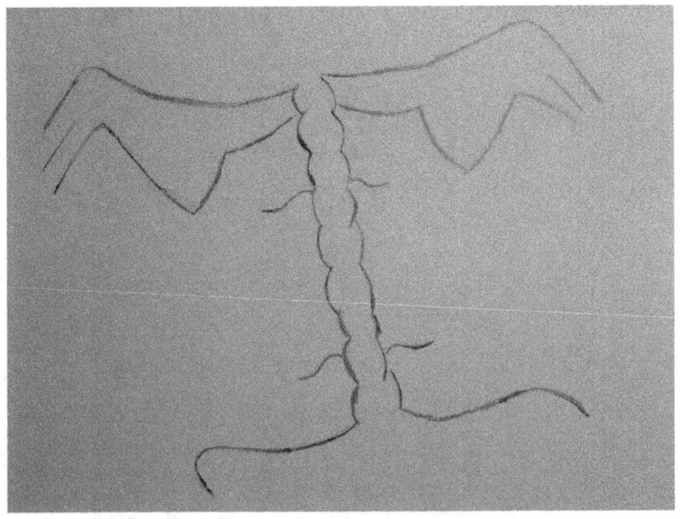

We developed a new set of exercises that would target this area in particular to activate the signals controlling it.

Holding onto the parallel bars to support his back, squats were a main exercise at this point. With him aiming every time he is getting up to keep his back as upright as possible. If he can't then I would put it into the right position for him.

It had to be upright, otherwise the exercise wouldn't be effective in the long term and he would be reliant on the areas we have developed rather than working on developing the paralysed core.

This seemed to be achieving what we were looking for. Gradually, his back was becoming less collapsible and when he sat down he wouldn't be falling over in any direction.

Still we needed to keep going for a long time to get him into a position where he would not be vulnerable in this area. But we were heading in the right direction.

The main things for us now was that he was no longer paralysed. His disability is for life but he is not paralysed with it. He is capable of taking part in activities he likes and overcoming his disability.

We have managed to significantly improve his quality of life.

21 SPEECH

With the twins difficulties, speech was a slow progress in the beginning. But with practice they were the first in their class to count to ten and to know the alphabet.

22 WRITING

Writing was something we had to work on for years for Noah, particularly as we worked on the setback by the wrong prescriptions with his eyes.

Initially his writing was all over the page with him trying to control his hold. We are still working on this now but it is much more legible than it used to be and keeps improving.

23 TAKING A STAND

We had been working on our new exercises targeting his core for nearly a year when he managed to take a stand unaided.

We had decided to go on holiday without his walking frame. And while we were away, he managed to take the first stand.

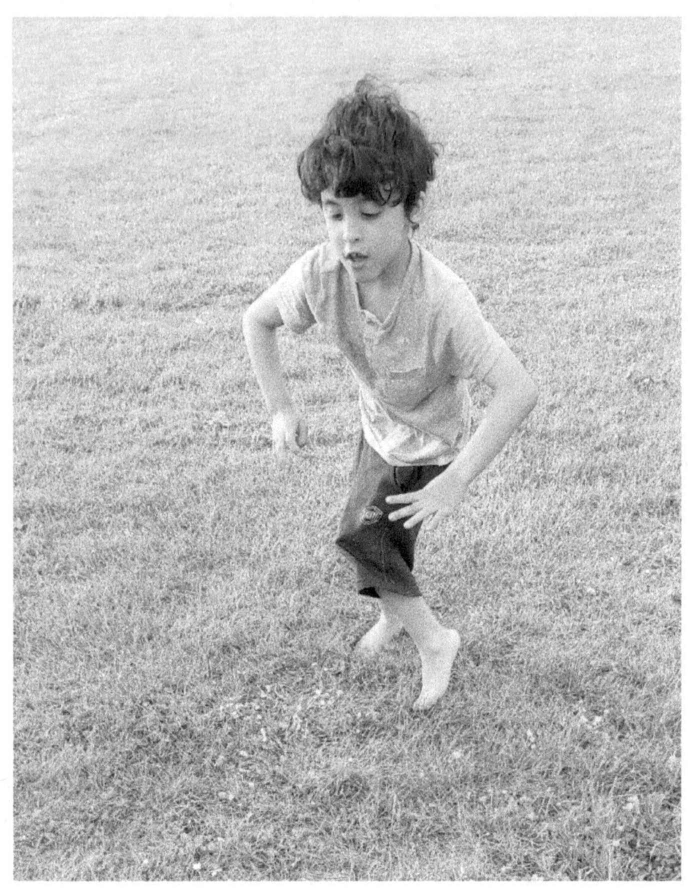

This was a nice surprise for all of us. It was evident that we had been doing all the right things.

When we came home, we continued practicing. He could stand just for a couple of seconds but we kept going at it.

55

How To Help Your Disabled Child

seconds but we kept going at it.

24 MILESTONE

Over a long period of time, his back had become stronger. Persistence with the exercises everyday and determination to achieve progress had yielded excellent results.

His back was no longer collapsible. It would not fall over in any direction like it used to. He could control his spine himself and hold it upright.

We had come a very long way since the days of needing a steel frame built around his spine in everyday activities. Even sitting down to have dinner was a problem at the time.

Now instead of collapsing completely, one would see a slight inclination in any direction.

We are still working on making all these muscles supporting his spine even stronger. But the main milestone at this point is that his spine is no longer vulnerable to collapsing anytime.

25 WALKING

With spine paralysis out of the way, taking some steps was a natural development that followed.

He could now control his back and keep it upright by using the muscles we have developed to support his spine. He could take a couple of steps at a time. Then these became some steps.

This was a very complex stage and involved many new developments of several parts of his body. There was his back which he was having to keep upright, there was his core which he was having to keep balanced to help the movement of his legs, there was his feet which he was having to keep in walking position, and his legs which had been reliant on his upper body in his walking frame and now they were having to carry the full weight of his body.

Nevertheless we still managed to make some progress and get all these things to function in synchrony in order for him to make some steps.

26 SPLINTS

Almost all children with cerebral palsy are prescribed something called splints, these are foot supports that are supposed to keep the ankles in good position. They are relevant in some cases but in Noah's they were more of a hindrance.

When he would try to get up on his own or do his walking practice whether in his walking frame or taking a few steps without it, these would dig in the back of his calves. Besides the fact that they do not support the natural walking movement and he had to lift his feet completely off the floor every time he needed to take steps in any direction.

We took them off completely and did

without. This was a decision we made after careful consideration of his walking development and fully exploring all our options. We went to every orthotics centre in Leeds and tried every type of splints available. I even imported European shoes with built-in splints but they had the same hindrance effects.

Boots were the way forward. Good boots would support his ankles and at the same time allow him the flexibility of the natural walking movements.

We also had to work on improving the footing of his steps so that they are not affecting his ankles in the wrong way.

I was pleased to see that the medical professionals agreed with us also on this occasion, seeing the difference we were managing to make without the prescribed splints.

27 NEW WALKING FRAME

We had been through a number of walking frames by then. Some of them were better than other. Some of them more practical and fold better. Some of them took too much space and were too difficult for him to operate.

The one he had recently got was okay and suitable for playing when he wanted to. But it had the same thing in common with previous walking frames. It relied too much on his upper body supporting his weight and dragging the weight of the frame behind him.

With our progress with his spine and his legs, it was time to get something different. The new walking frame had a higher point of hold, and a foldable seat within it, and it was a push one. This keeps all his body weight on his legs, and at the same time allows him to support his core by holding on. When he is tired after some steps he can put the seat down and take a break for a bit.

We went trick or treating in it last Halloween, and he was very happy being able to do that like other children. He had been trick or treating in it before but he had to be pushed all the time. This time he could go in it for his trick or treat and be pushed in-between.

28 EPILOGUE

I was putting his boots on in the morning before going to school, but his toes kept overlapping.

'Noah, don't do that!'
'I am not daddy. It's just that every time I try to move my toes nothing happens.'

This was how everything was in the beginning. He had quadruple paralysis as part of his cerebral palsy. An injury that was not his fault from the beginning.

It has taken us ten years to get to this point.

He can now stand and he can take some steps, he can take part in some activities and sports as he wishes.

We could have reached this point sooner, had we had a stable life with less problems. Our Reflective Signalling was also new and had never been done before. Every step we made in every direction was something innovative that we were trying for the first time for us and for humanity.

Noah's disability is for life but his paralysis is not.

Our journey continues with fine tuning many of the skills Noah had developed, getting him stronger and healthier as the days go by, and working on minor areas like his toes and his fingers.

We hope by writing this book in a simple and down to earth language to have provided an everyday guide for any person with someone in their life who suffers from the condition. And we hope that all children who suffer from cerebral palsy could find in this guide a way to improve the quality of their lives and becoming more independent every day.

29 THE TICKLES

In the final stages of preparing this book for publication we have had some movement in the toes. We had only been working on new exercises targeting this area for a few weeks. So this was a good surprise.

Other areas of his body took us years and this is including his legs. But targeting areas such as the toes is mainly fine tuning a part of his body that has been generally developed over many years.

The development of feeling his toes has

also given him the tickles on a number of occasions, and particularly before bed. We all laugh with him.

ABOUT THE AUTHOR

H Bastawy came to existence in Alexandria to parents who were practically foreign to the culture they were living in. His father could trace his ancestry at least from one parent to an African country that does not exist today, and his mother had ancestral heritage that went back to the days of Russian monarchy, a political system that also does not exist today. He could not be born like other people, after ten months of his conception they decided to try to get him out somehow. His mother expected a girl and planned to call him Heidi, or Horace for a boy. Horace was not a name that could be pronounced in the environment that they were in, so they named him Haythem which is a variation of that name. He prefers H instead which is a more neutral name – being gender neutral himself - and the initial for all these names across all these languages. He went to a European school and he grew up as an Englishman, with English being his first language. In his childhood and teens he took to music, drama and sports, he also liked philosophy and invented some things. He had a keyboard and a guitar, and he played them fairly well, taking part in music festivals and concerts. He did not attend school very much, partly because of having to go on many trips winning championships and tournaments, but mainly because he got really bored. Despite not going to school, he managed to obtain many degrees as an adult. He does not however count his BA because it was certified by corrupt officials through a corrupt process. He is generally known as H, or Dr/Professor Bastawy. He is Anglican Christian (this means Church of England), with some Jewish and pagan heritage. However he is not religious and has never been. He lives and works from home in Leeds, England, with his children. Him and his children are so young that sometimes they get mistaken for brothers and sisters. He spent some of his earlier years as an agent in military intelligence.

H Bastawy is a multi-award winning author and artist. His rock albums have attracted worldwide attention. Some of his songs were featured on TV and many of his stories were featured in movies. He is World number 1 in Academia worldwide author ranking. www.HBastawy.com

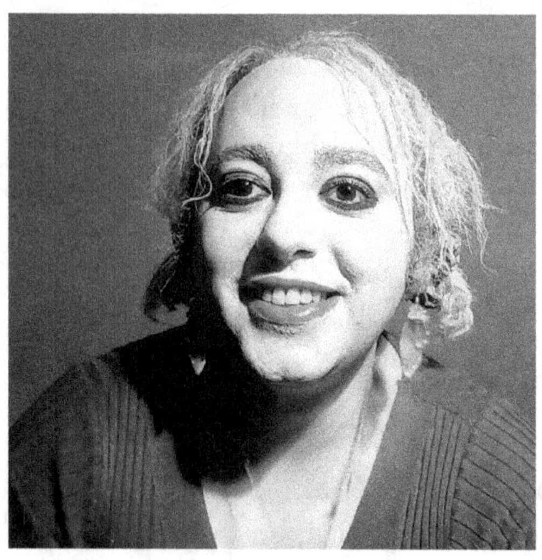

9 798323 210084